How to Lower High Blood Pressure using Cayenne Pepper

NIGEL THOMAS

Published by Samoht Publishing
samohtpublishing@mail.com

Copyright © 2013 Samoht Publishing

ISBN-10: 1484072650
ISBN-13: 978-1484072653

Cover Photo Acknowledgement
pushbeyond from stock.xchng

DEDICATION

This book is dedicated to all those who seek an alternative way of treating their health issues.

I wish you all a long and healthy life.

CONTENTS

ACKNOWLEDGMENTS

I would like to acknowledge all the help and encouragement my wife Jane has given me in the writing of this book, I would also like to thank my daughter Claire for her support.

Without these two in my life this book would probably never have been written.

INTRODUCTION

High blood pressure is something we all experience from time to time. If you take part in any physical exercise, get stressed or angry, your blood pressure will rise. This is normal, there is nothing wrong with that so long as it returns back to normal after a short period of time.

When it becomes a problem though, is when your blood pressure remains high for any length of time.

Blood pressure refers to the force of blood against the walls of the arteries. When blood pressure remains elevated over any period of time it is called high blood pressure, or hypertension.

It is a sad fact that hypertension is on the increase these days, in truth more people suffer from high blood pressure now than at any other time.

This is mainly due to the sedate lifestyle and modern eating habits that the majority of us have adopted.

It is estimated that in the UK alone almost one third of adults have high blood pressure. That is an alarming statistic!

But, what is even more alarming is the fact that many of them don't even know they have it.

This is why high blood pressure is sometimes called the silent killer, because there are no real symptoms for people to pick up on. Some people, the lucky ones, might suffer from a lot of headaches which may eventually get diagnosed as high blood pressure by their doctor.

But the majority of us go about our daily lives totally oblivious to the fact that we are suffering from high blood pressure.

But make no mistake, high blood pressure really is a killer if not detected and controlled.

How do I know if my blood pressure is high?

You can probably remember times when you have visited your doctor and he has strapped on an inflatable band around your upper arm. This is how he checks your blood pressure. If he finds it is higher or lower than normal he will ask you to come back over the next couple of days to have it checked again.

This is because our blood pressure can fluctuate at different times and needs to be checked over a couple of days.

So, this is how most people learn they have high blood pressure. But, of course, there are a lot of people who do not visit their doctor on a regular basis.

Visiting an optician for an eye test can also reveal you have high blood pressure. But, once again, not everyone will have regular eye tests.

These are the people most at risk of having high blood pressure and never realizing it!

What is considered to be high blood pressure?

When your doctor takes your blood pressure he measures the maximum pressure (systolic) and the lowest pressure (diastolic) of the beating of the heart.

Normal blood pressure shows a reading of 120/70 mm Hg. If the reading shows a measurement between 120/80 mm Hg and 139/89 mm Hg then you have what is known as pre hypertension.

High blood pressure is described as anything showing a reading of 140/90 mm Hg or above.

What is pre hypertension?

It means that at this particular moment in time you do not have high blood pressure, but are considered likely to develop it in the future.

Even for those who have managed to reach the age of 55 without having high blood pressure still stand a 90 percent chance of developing it later in their lifetime.

High blood pressure is a condition that most people will have at some point in their lives.

Obviously this means it is important to learn all you can about it and, more importantly, to learn what can be done to keep your blood pressure at the right level.

This is where cayenne pepper becomes so important with regards to high blood pressure.

Read on to learn more.

EFFECTS OF HIGH BLOOD PRESSURE

When your blood pressure is high the effects on your body are focused on four main areas: Eyes, Kidneys, Arteries and Heart.

Eyes – High blood pressure can cause the blood vessels in your eyes to burst and lead to eye disease. This is called Hypertensive Retinopathy and the damage this causes can be very serious if not treated. Symptoms can include headaches and impaired vision.

As mentioned before, an optician can detect high blood pressure when carrying out an eye test so it is important to have your eyes checked regularly to make sure you do not go on to develop Hypertension Retinopathy.

Kidneys – As you would expect the kidneys are important to your overall health and wellbeing. They are made up of tiny blood vessels that act as a filter to expel the wastes from your blood and body.

As with most conditions of high blood pressure it is something of a catch twenty-two situation where the kidneys are concerned.

A hormone is produced by a healthy kidney to help regulate its own blood pressure.

But, high blood pressure can cause the tiny blood vessels in your kidneys to thicken and narrow meaning they cannot function as well as they would normally, resulting in less waste being filtered from your blood.

As the kidney becomes more and more unhealthy it is no longer able to regulate its blood pressure which then causes your blood pressure to increase even more. Hence the catch twenty-two situation.

More worryingly, it can also cause your kidneys to fail altogether.

If that were to happen you would need to go on dialysis every couple of days or even have a kidney transplant.

Those people who´s blood pressure is found to be high will almost certainly have a test carried out on their kidneys too, as the two go hand in hand together.

Arteries – High blood pressure will exert greater pressure on the walls of your arteries which can in turn create microscopic tears which then heal as scar tissue.

The scar tissue can then become a magnet for attracting plaques such as fat and cholesterol. As this plaque builds up over time the artery becomes narrower and hardened meaning less blood can pass along it. This can cause conditions such as peripheral artery disease and coronary artery disease.

When the arteries have become narrowed by plaque and fatty deposits there is a greater chance of a blood clot forming. These blood clots are then carried around in your blood stream until they become lodged and either partly or completely stop the blood supply altogether.

As the damaged arteries fail to supply the right amount of blood to your body´s organs, these organs also begin to fail , adding to your problems.

Heart – Obviously, if the particular organ that is being starved of oxygen carrying blood is the heart, then this can lead to serious, if not live threatening, problems.

When not enough oxygen reaches the heart, then a chest pain known as Angina can develop.

When the heart cannot receive enough blood

because of blocked arteries then a heart attack can develop.

High blood pressure is the number one risk factor for congestive heart failure. This is where the heart is unable to pump enough blood around to the rest of the body.

Additional information – Although I have said earlier that high blood pressure is focused on four main areas of the body, there is of course one other area that needs to be considered, if you are a man that is.

Once the flow of blood through the arteries has become blocked or weakened it will become increasingly more difficult for a man to reach his full sexual potential. It will eventually lead to him suffering from erectile dysfunction, or impotency as it is more commonly known.

A NATURAL CURE FOR HIGH BLOOD PRESSURE

The usual approach to getting your blood pressure down is for your doctor to prescribe you a series of medications or tablets.

Although each person is different, the aim of the medication is to get you to reach a target level of around 140/90 mm Hg if you are under the age of 80, and a slightly higher target of around 150/90 mm Hg for older patients.

For those who have gone on to suffer from cardiovascular disease, kidney disease or diabetes their target will be set to around the 130/80 mm Hg or below.

There are five main classes of medication that are

prescribed to lower blood pressure. They are as follows:

Angiotensin-converting enzyme (ACE) inhibitors

With brand names such as - captopril, cilazapril, enalapril, fosinopril, lisinopril, perindopril, quinapril, ramipril, and trandolapril.

Angiotensin receptor blockers

With brand names such as - candesartan, eprosartan, irbesartan, losartan, olmesartan, telmisartan and valsartan.

Calcium-channel blockers

With brand names such as - amlodipine, diltiazem, felodipine, isradipine, lacidipine, lercanidipine, nicardipine, nifedipine, nisoldipine, and verapamil.

Diuretics (water tablets)

With brand names such as - bendroflumethiazide, chlorothiazide, chlortalidone, cyclopenthiazide, hydrochlorothiazide and indapamide.

Beta-blockers

With brand names such as - acebutolol, atenolol, bisoprolol, metoprolol, oxprenolol, pindolol, propranolol, sotalol, and timolol.

Unfortunately, as with most medicines, there are often side-effects to taking these medications.

For instance:

Ace inhibitors – can sometimes cause an irritating cough.

Angiotensin receptor blockers – can sometimes cause dizziness.

Calcium-channel blockers – can sometimes cause dizziness, facial flushing, constipation and swollen ankles.

Diuretics – can sometimes cause gout, or for those who already have gout make it worse, as well as developing impotence for some users.

Beta-blockers – can sometimes cause users to suffer cold hands and feet, tiredness with poor sleep and impotence for some users.

As you can see, the big drug companies *(see Drug Companies)* have certainly latched onto a money making opportunity here. Not only do they make and sell the drugs in the first place but they then have a ready made market to sell another drug to counter-act the side-effects of the first one.

But, instead of suffering the possible side-effect of these medications, why not try an alternative?

A word of caution here! Before making any dramatic changes to your medications I would seriously advise speaking to your doctor first!

Better still, for those who do not yet suffer from high blood pressure but want to ensure they never do, why not start taking this alternative product as a preventative.

Because this product is not only natural and free from any additives but is often called a miracle cure.

You won't find this particular product on a drug store shelf though. You will though, more probably, find it in your local health food shop or maybe even at the back of your kitchen cupboard.

Because the natural product we are talking about is cayenne pepper!

And this really does have the right to be called *a miracle cure.*

So what's so good about cayenne pepper?

For hundreds of years cayenne pepper, or Capsicum as it is sometimes also known, has been used as not only flavouring for meals but also for its many different health benefits. These health benefits are far to numerous to mention here *(see Benefits at a Glance)* but trust me when I say they range from the digestive system, the heart and blood vessels, the prostate, and many other major organs too.

In fact cayenne pepper is well known for fortifying the overall health of your entire body.

And the good news for you is that it is also fantastic at lowering high blood pressure.

HOW TO USE CAYENNE PEPPER

C ayenne pepper can be taken either as a drink or applied onto the skin as an ointment, depending on what condition you want to treat. But in the case of a high blood pressure we are going to take it as a drink.

Cayenne pepper can be bought in two different forms, either as a powder or a capsule. It is very much dependent on personal preference as to which form you buy. Both have their merits.

Myself, I prefer to take cayenne pepper in the powdered form. This is simply because I find it easier, if needed, to adjust the amount of cayenne I use. And I also find the powder absorbs into the blood stream quicker which means it takes less time to feel its benefits.

So for this reason the following methods use powdered cayenne.

How to use cayenne pepper in a drink

The thing to bear in mind here is that cayenne pepper is very hot, and if you take too much it can actually make you vomit. So the sensible thing is to start slowly with small amounts to allow your body to get used to it.

The preparation for the drink is very simple.

Add the cayenne pepper powder to a cup or glass, pour the required amount of hot water over the cayenne then let it rest for a minute. Stir the mixture well so that as much of the cayenne is absorbed into the liquid and then drink.

You may find it best to either continue stirring, or swirling, the mixture as you drink it to ensure the cayenne doesn't sink to the bottom of the cup.

Listed next are the various recipes for using cayenne pepper to treat or help lower high blood pressure.

CAYENNE FOR LOWERING HIGH BLOOD PRESSURE

You may well be asking yourself why is cayenne pepper so good at lowering high blood pressure? Well that is a good question, and hopefully you will begin to see its merits as you read on.

Scientific research has now proved what many others have known for years that Cayenne pepper, or Spanish pepper, American red pepper, African red pepper, capsicum, and bird pepper as it is also known, can create a positive effect and improvement on the cardiovascular system.

It has the ability to stop an heart attack, remove plaque from the arteries and generally nourish the heart with vital nutrients.

Cayenne pepper is known to improve the overall health of your heart by improving circulation, lowering cholesterol, rebuilding blood cells, emulsifying triglycerides, and removing toxins such as arterial plaque from your bloodstream making the blood flow more smoothly.

More importantly from our point of view, when taken with hot water cayenne can also equalize your blood pressure by regulating the flow of blood from your head to your feet.

Let's see how we can go about this by making a cayenne pepper tea.

Cayenne Pepper Tea

Ingredients:

4 ounces (120 ml) of boiling water - let it cool a little first

¼ teaspoon cayenne pepper powder, increasing to ½ tsp

½ teaspoon of honey

Firstly put the cayenne pepper powder into a cup along with the honey, heat a kettle of water to just below boiling, then measure out the water and pour it into the cup.

Stir until all the ingredients are mixed together well.

As you drink the mixture keep stirring, or swilling the cup, so that the cayenne powder doesn't sink to the bottom and give you a nasty surprise with the last mouthful.

Take once each and every day.

This is a good recipe to start off with, and one that I take on a daily basis.

It will begin to lower your blood pressure if it is high but it is also a very good recipe to prevent your blood pressure getting high in the first place.

If you find this amount of cayenne a little too hard to cope with at first, then you might want to reduce the amount of cayenne pepper a little or increase the amount of water to 8 ounces (240 ml).

I have also found that shop bought honey has a much lower strength than organic honey. So the amount in this recipe is also something that you can adjust to suit your taste.

Depending on how high your blood pressure is you will eventually want to increase the amount you take to ½ a teaspoon of cayenne pepper powder with the above recipe to give you maximum benefit.

If you blood pressure is really stubborn you can even increase the cayenne pepper powder to 1 teaspoon with the recipes both above and below.

A word of warning here though, don't go for the larger amount too soon. Believe me you won't thank yourself for going to quickly.

Let your body tell you when it is okay to up the dose.

With regards to the water. If you have to blow on the water before you can drink it, and then have to sip it, then the water is too hot. You want it to be somewhere between warm and boiling. Ideally you will be able to swallow a mouthful at a time.

Cayenne Pepper with Tomato Juice

Ingredients:

4 ounces (120 ml) of tomato juice

¼ teaspoon cayenne pepper powder, increasing to ½ tsp

Mix all the ingredients together and drink once a day. As before, when you feel ready, increase the cayenne pepper to ½ teaspoon, or if needed even 1 whole teaspoon.

You can also use any other juice you like but tomato juice does seem to help with high blood pressure.

If you are having a regular blood pressure test you should begin to see your levels drop within a week or so.

HOW TO PREVENT
HIGH BLOOD PRESSURE

T his book has primarily been concerned with lowering blood pressure that has already reached a high level.

As you will already have read, high blood pressure can, if left untreated, have very serious effects on your health and lifestyle. Especially if you are unaware that it has already reached a high level

That is, after all, why it has become known as the silent killer!

So, in my opinion, prevention is better than a cure! Let's face it, it must be better to do all you can to keep your blood pressure normal, than to sit back and do nothing at all.

This is something that cayenne pepper is ideally suited to doing for you. Even if you take the cayenne pepper tea recipe with just a ¼ teaspoon of cayenne, on a daily basis, then the benefits will begin to pay off in no time.

As you have already read, your blood pressure will become equalized from your head to your feet, your cholesterol levels will begin to fall, toxins will be removed from your bloodstream and your blood will begin to flow more smoothly.

That sounds like a pretty good way of staving off the onset of high blood pressure to me, and all without the accompanying side-effects of blood pressure drugs.

It might well be worth investing in a home blood pressure test kit. Some of these are now quite inexpensive and can be bought in your local pharmacist or drug store and even at Amazon.com.

Please though, do read the instruction manual with regards to how and when to take your blood pressure. And remember, from time to time your blood pressure fluctuates naturally so don't be over alarmed if at times you see it rise a little. This is why it needs to be checked over a number of days. Consult your manual regarding this.

Other ways to prevent high blood pressure

Exercise will obviously have a beneficial effect on

keeping your blood pressure down. The word "exercise" often conjures up an image of spending hours in a gym building up a sweat. But this really doesn't have to be the case.

Light, simple exercise is all that is needed, nothing too strenuous. Walking is a good form of exercise, not a stroll or an amble, but a reasonably paced walk for twenty minutes to half an hour is all that it take. Taking the dog for a walk is more or less all it would take. And if you don´t own a dog of your own, borrow one.

It is also very good for getting your weight down.

And for those who need to, shedding a few pounds will also help keep your blood pressure down. Because without doubt, those who are overweight stand a greater chance of also suffering with high blood pressure.

You might remember I mentioned the catch twenty two situation before? Well the more overweight you are the more chance of your blood pressure being high. The higher your blood pressure, the more chance of it increasing.

Eat healthily! I am sure people often wonder to themselves what that statement means.

Well in its crudest form, think of whatever meals you like and stop eating them! Only joking, well partially anyway.

A healthy diet doesn't consist of junk food, not on a daily basis anyway. These are the sort of meals that will, over time, begin to block up your arteries with cholesterol, make you overweight and cause your blood pressure to increase.

To eat more healthily try and cut out as much fat as you can, keep red meat down to about one portion a week, cut back on alcohol to around one drink a day and above all, stop smoking.

A quick search on the internet will give you plenty of pointers about eating a healthy diet and adopting a healthier lifestyle.

So to sum up, regularly take a tonic that will have overall beneficial effects on your body and cardiovascular system, such as cayenne pepper tea, take regular exercise and adopt a healthier diet.

FREQUENTLY ASKED QUESTIONS

Which is best, the capsule or powder?

That is really down to your own preference, but in my opinion I prefer cayenne pepper as a powder. This is simply because I use different amount to treat different symptoms and I find the powder absorbs into my blood stream quicker.

How often should I take cayenne pepper?

This really depends on what symptoms you are taking cayenne pepper for. With regards to high blood pressure see the recipes in this book.

When should I take cayenne pepper?

You can take cayenne pepper anytime of the day that suits you. There are, however, times when it is advisable not to take cayenne pepper. I would avoid taking after a heavy meal, and certainly neither before or after any strenuous exercise.

How hot should the drink be?

Once again this depends on what you are taking cayenne pepper for. But generally speaking if you are taking the powder with water then the heat of the water is best somewhere between hot and boiling. Although if you are taking it with a juice then obviously it can be taken cold.

Is cayenne powder from a supermarket okay?

Yes it is, but you won't get the best result from using this variety. The reason for this is because it will more than likely have been irradiated. This is basically done to give it a longer shelf life, but in doing so it loses some of its potency.

The supermarket variety of cayenne powder is more suitable to be used as a spice to add flavor to food such as curries. That is not to say that you won't get any benefit from this but it will be limited.

Where is the best place to buy cayenne powder?

The best place to buy cayenne powder would be from your local health food shop, or from an herbal wholesalers on-line website. You can even buy cayenne pepper powder from Amazon.com

Which is the best cayenne powder to buy?

Cayenne is actually ranked by measuring the levels

of capsaicin it contains. There are two methods of measuring these levels, the Gillette Method and the Scoville Heat Units (SHU). The Scoville measuring scale has become the most popular method.

Cayenne is rated from 30,000 to 50,000 SHUs. That is the rate I would recommend starting with, and all the recipes in this book use this rate.

If you look in your local health food shop, or online, you will find cayenne that is hotter than this. In fact it can go right up to 140,000 SHUs which, as you can imagine, is extremely hot.

But, I would not recommend buying cayenne rated any higher than 50,000SHUs until you are completely comfortable with that level of heat.

The old saying "buyer beware" is very apt with this situation.

Will cayenne pepper make me feel ill?

Taking cayenne pepper powder as a drink will certainly make your lips, mouth and tongue feel warm or have a very slight burning sensation.

If you drink cayenne after any strenuous exercise you might well end up with a bad stomachache.

But, if you take a large amount in one go it could make you vomit!

Read the instructions in this book about starting small and building up the amount of cayenne you take.

Does cayenne pepper taste nice?

Taste is very subjective, so that's difficult to answer. Cayenne pepper has a very pungent taste which some people might like while others won't. At best, I would say it is an acquired taste that has a lot of very beneficial qualities.

OTHER HEALTH BENEFITS OF CAYENNE PEPPER

A s you read through this list of benefits you will begin to see why it was no exaggeration when I called cayenne pepper a miracle cure.

Heart and Cardiovascular

Cayenne is able to equalize the body's blood pressure by regulating the flow of blood from the head to the feet. This has an obviously beneficial effect on not only the heart itself, but also to the arteries, capillaries and nerves too.

Cholesterol can be lowered with regular use of cayenne pepper, it is also beneficial for all forms of heart disease, as well as preventing and treating blood clots.

It has been claimed that cayenne pepper can even stop an heart attack in its tracks.

Digestive System

Cayenne is very good at promoting digestion by stimulating the flow of saliva and enabling a feeble stomach to digest food more easily.

It is also very good for the treatment of heartburn, dyspepsia and flatulence due to its carminative effect.

It can also aid the digestive system by rebuilding the tissues in the stomach to help heal the stomach and stomach ulcers.

Because cayenne pepper produces a natural feeling of warmth in your body this stimulates the motion of the intestines to help with the assimilation and elimination.

When used in larger quantities (above 20g) cayenne can be used as a laxative to induce frequent bowel movements.

Cayenne can also be used for relieving sea-sickness too.

Immune System

Cayenne can help improve the whole immune system by alleviating allergies and muscle cramps and helping wounds to heal more quickly and without as much scarring.

It can also help ease the pain of rheumatism and arthritis, joint pains and swellings, as well chronic lumbago too.

Cayenne is good at helping to improve the health of the body's vital organs such as the kidney, spleen and pancreas. It can also be used to stimulate the gall bladder reflex.

When taken internally it is particularly good at treating the symptoms of colds as its warming effect has a powerful action on the mucous membrane.

Cancers

An article in the journal Cancer Research, reports on a study carried out by Dr Soren Lehmann of the Cedars-Sinai Medical Center in Los Angeles where he claims that the main ingredient in cayenne, capsaicin, was able to destroy cancer cells in the prostate.

He said, "Capsaicin led 80 percent of human prostate cancer cells, growing in mice, to commit suicide in a process known as apoptosis."

The study revealed that prostate cancer tumors in mice fed on capsaicin were about one-fifth the size of tumors in untreated mice.

BENEFITS AT A GLANCE

Stops heart attack instantly

Lowers blood pressure

Lowers cholesterol

Re-builds blood cells

Clears out arteries

Removes toxins from blood stream

Kills prostate cancer cells

Helps recover from frostbite

Heals Hemorrhoids

Re-builds stomach tissue

Heals stomach ulcers

Improves circulation

Improves digestion

Relieves heartburn and indigestion

Soothes toothache

Relieves fever

Relieves a sore throat

Helps to ease and reduce a cough

Eases osteoarthritis and rheumatoid pain

Helps relieve shingles

Eases joint pains

Used as a laxative

Used to stop diarrhea

Heals cuts and wounds

Helps relieve malaria

SIDE EFFECTS AND WARNINGS

T he main thing to stress here is that cayenne pepper has very few side-effect like pharmaceutical drugs but, like anything beneficial, needs to be taken in moderation. It is also wise to start with a smaller dose and gradually build up to the required amount to avoid any discomfort.

Cayenne pepper is often taken as a powder, a pill or even whole. It can also be used as an ointment directly onto the skin.

When you first start taking cayenne pepper as a drink in its powdered form you will notice a warming or mild burning of the lips, mouth and throat.

This is normal and should last for only a couple of minutes at the most.

Skin and eye irritation

After using powdered cayenne make sure to wash your hands thoroughly as any contact to the eyes can cause very bad irritation. I can personally testify to this! Be careful using it on your skin as an ointment as those with sensitive skin may find it can burn or itch.

Allergic Reaction

Before taking cayenne pepper it is best to check that you are not likely to suffer from an allergic reaction to it. Those people who are already allergic to chestnuts, latex, kiwis, avocados or bananas are more likely to be allergic to cayenne too.

The symptoms of cayenne allergy may include difficulty breathing, swelling of the throat, vomiting, hives and loss of consciousness. If you begin to suffer any of these symptoms after taking cayenne ***seek medical help urgently.***

Gastrointestinal upset

Although cayenne pepper is in most cases a benefit to the digestive system for some people it may cause a mild irritation of the stomach. This is often because too big a dose was taken in one go.

The way around this is to start with a small amount and slowly build up the dosage until you arrive at the desired amount.

It is also wise not to take cayenne pepper straight

after doing any strenuous form of exercise as this will also cause you to suffer from stomach ache.

Other issues

It is not advisable to administer cayenne to children under the age of two.

If you are breastfeeding do not take cayenne orally.

If you are pregnant do not take cayenne without first consulting with your doctor.

Do not take large doses for any long periods of time as this can cause damage to your liver and kidneys.

Stop using at least two weeks before any surgery as cayenne can cause increased bleeding.

If you are taking any prescribed medication consult your doctor before using cayenne pepper as the capsicum in this herb can clash with other drugs.

DRUG COMPANIES

Having just read all about the amazing health qualities of cayenne peppers you are probably wondering why this knowledge isn't more widely known.

The truth is it's because the big drug companies don't want you to know. They make a lot of money from manufacturing and selling medicines because there is a lot of money to be made from health products. Or, to put it more accurately from products for ill-health.

So, you can see, it is not in their interest for you to know about other, often much cheaper, methods and products to relieve your illness.

And to some point that is quite understandable. The pharmaceutical industry employs huge numbers of highly trained scientists and technical staff to run their business. Their research and development budgets are massive and obviously all those costs have to be passed onto someone. Normally the end user – which is you!

So it is only natural that having made such a huge up-front investment they don't want people to know of other methods of finding a cure to their illness.

The other point to bear in mind here too, is that the pharmaceutical industry is actually a chemical industry. The end result is a drug, or chemical, that you ingest in your body.

And as we all know these drugs or chemicals can, and do, have their side effects.

For example. A couple of years back I came across a copy of the US edition of the Reader Digest, rather than the UK edition (now no longer published) that I was used to reading.

There was just something about this edition that seemed odd to me, although I couldn't put my finger on it at first.

It wasn't until flipping through the pages a good few times that I realized what the difference was.

Throughout the UK edition there would be pages of articles and stories separated by the odd page or two of adverts.

But in the US edition it was slightly different. It also had all the pages of articles and stories, just like the UK edition, but when it featured an advert for a medical product, like lets say indigestion tablets, there followed two or three full pages of disclaimers.

The disclaimers were in such small type I had to strain my eyes to simply read them.

As America has more of a claims culture than the UK these pages were there to warn the consumer all about the different side effects of this particular product.

Page after page!

In the case of the indigestion tablets it even warned you that you could suffer with – wait for it – indigestion.

So what is the point of buying a product that the makers know, along with all its other side effects, could give you the very thing you are taking it to try and cure.

Absolute madness!

And yet it is these sort of products the majority of us turn to each and every time we want to relieve the symptom of our particular ailment.

Surely it is much better, for your body as well as your health, to use a natural product rather than a more chemical based one?

CONCLUSION

Thank you for buying and reading How to Lower High Blood Pressure with Cayenne Pepper.

I am sure you will find the information contained within this book to be fascinating, and that you will look at the fiery red hot cayenne pepper in a completely different light from now on.

I can honestly say that if you follow the advice and directions given within these pages you will quickly discover why I am so enthusiastic about using cayenne pepper.

As someone who takes cayenne pepper on a daily basis I can personally testify to its benefits as can so many others who regularly use it too.

If you have enjoyed reading this book and found the information helpful I would be grateful if you would add a review of it so other people might benefit from it also.

Thank you,

Nigel Thomas

OTHER BOOKS BY THIS PUBLISHER

The books listed below can be found at Amazon in their Kindle section.

Cayenne Pepper Health Benefits

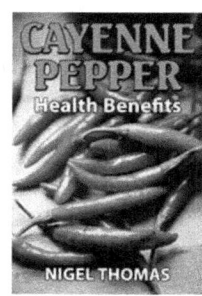 I have written this book as a follow on from my other two successful books on Cayenne Pepper - *Cure Sore Throats, Colds and Coughs with Cayenne Pepper* and *How to Lower High Blood Pressure using Cayenne Pepper.* I decided to write this book because I realised so many people were looking for a more natural way to treat their health problems.

That is why I have tried to show you all the different benefits that can be found in cayenne pepper. Or as Dr.

Richard Schulze, the famed medical herbalist put it, -

"If you master only one herb in your life, master cayenne pepper. It is more powerful than any other."

In this book you will learn how cayenne pepper can help heal such ailments as -

Blood Pressure, Arthritis, Allergies, Sinusitis, Tooth Ache . . . and even Cancer

I have included recipes for the different doses and mixtures and have even included a chapter on making your own cayenne infused oil and cayenne tincture.

Cure Sore Throats, Colds and Coughs with Cayenne Pepper

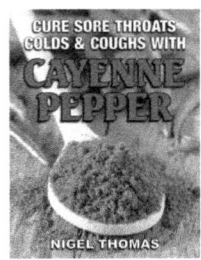

Once the sore throat and aching limbs of a cold begin, what you need is something that will quickly relieve the symptoms and get you back onto the road to recovery. Cayenne pepper is the very thing.

Although there are many over the counter products that claim to be able to do this, cayenne pepper is a natural product that has a huge healing benefit.

Learn how using this secret miracle cure will relieve the symptoms of a cold quickly and easily.

Miracle is not a work used lightly to describe the healing benefits of Cayenne Pepper.

This book describes in detail the usage and directions for each step to cure a sore throat, cold and cough.

41

For anyone wanting a more natural approach to recover from a cold or flu like symptoms then Cayenne Pepper should be at the top of your list.

In this book you will learn:

The different recipes and dosages to be taken for each stage of the cold.

The benefits and reasons why they help you . . .

. . . and, how often to use them.

The healing properties of this natural spice should not be taken lightly, its benefits go way beyond just relieving a cold or flu and these benefits are also listed in this book.

Affirmations for Health, Wealth and Happiness

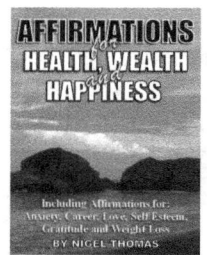

We are all looking for health, wealth and happiness - but few of us ever find it. Probably because we don't know how to go about finding it.

But this illustrated book of affirmations will teach you how!

I am sure you have all heard of affirmations before, maybe even used one or two over the years, but did you ever realize how important affirmations are and the effect they have on you?

In this book you will learn:

Why affirmations are so important.

What positive affirmations are.

Why you should use them.

How often to use them . . .

. . . and, find examples of affirmations you can use for health, wealth and happiness, plus also affirmations for anxiety, career, love, self-esteem, gratitude and weight loss.

This is a GREAT little guide book of affirmations.

Earn Extra Money with a Sandwich Delivery Business

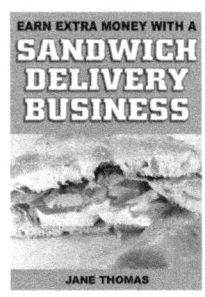

If you are looking to start a new business, or just want to earn some extra regular cash, then Earn Extra Money with a Sandwich Delivery Business is just the book you have been looking for.

Whether you are looking for a low start up business to give you a little extra money at the end of each month or something that will provide you with a full-time income - whilst only working part-time hours - then this is definitely a business you will want to look into.

I have run a successful sandwich delivery business for many years and in my book I explain exactly how to set up and run one for yourself.

Reading my book you will learn:

How to research your area

What licenses and permits you will need . . .

. . . and how to go about getting them

How to calculate your profit margin

What items you will need to get started

How to start and run either a Door to door, or Made to order sandwich business

How to keep a record of sales and expenditure

Plus, I even give you a list of tried and tested sandwich recipes, along with recipes for soups and cakes too.

Grab a copy of my book and learn how you to could Earn Extra Money with a Sandwich Delivery Business.

Read what people are saying about this book:

"This guide covers all the steps needed to open a sandwich delivery business. It even gives a brief overview of the authorities you need to get in contact with for licenses and permits, both in the UK & the US.

Most people jump into a business without conducting proper market research and doing the math. The author explains in great detail on these matters which to me are of utmost importance before you 'dive in'.

I recommend this book to anyone looking to open a food delivery or catering business."